I0118158

LET IT GO
Voices from the Deep

Kinshuk Sharma

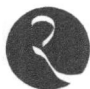

RUPA

Published by
Rupa Publications India Pvt. Ltd 2013
7/16, Ansari Road, Daryaganj
New Delhi 110002

Sales centres:
Allahabad Bengaluru Chennai
Hyderabad Jaipur Kathmandu
Kolkata Mumbai

Copyright © Kinshuk Sharma 2013

All rights reserved.
No part of this publication may be reproduced, transmitted,
or stored in a retrieval system, in any form or by any means, electronic,
mechanical, photocopying, recording or otherwise, without the prior
permission of the publisher.

ISBN 978-81-2912-983-3

First impression 2013

10 9 8 7 6 5 4 3 2 1

The moral right of the author has been asserted.

Printed at Repro Knowledgecast Limited, Thane

This book is sold subject to the condition that it shall not, by way
of trade or otherwise, be lent, resold, hired out, or otherwise circulated,
without the publisher's prior consent, in any form of binding or cover other
than that in which it is published.

To my Nana Ji
Dr Mathura Dutt Pandey,
for inspiring me to write

CONTENTS

HINDI SONGS

FOREWORD

The value of the limitless beauty of nature is surrounded by questions like who, what, why etc. No one can explain this whole plethora with words. But an emotional heart still cannot help but try, because though such incomparable beauty, overwhelming calmness, unstoppable feelings, fragrance etc. is soothing even at the outside, for an emotional man it initiates a wave of exploration and his poetic heart starts searching for that heartbeat that regular eyes cannot see. That is how his poetic journey starts which I have sculptured in the following lines:

> There's a flood of feelings in my heart
> That flowed through voice: became a song
> Some overflowed right through my eyes
> And that is where my heart belongs

The question is, why does an emotional man get sucked into that wave, by such exorbitant beauty which most others just enjoy? I believe that the emotional man gets connected to the view, in a sense that is larger than everything, even than him. His soul gets a flash through its subconscious from its past, from the ultimate.

This poet, in his early years of life, sits next to the ocean, alone, observes the coming and going of the sea waves, talks to the waves, listens to them but sometimes is not able to understand exactly what the waves have to say to him. He observes the race of waves, of time, but I wonder till where? Till the shore where only he is present? So, do the waves come to meet him there? If they do, then why do they leave? I believe that's when the storm hits the waves in his heart and such words flow from his pen:

The wave of love is leaving, but I'm glad I still see you
If you run into the sea, then, as sand I'd run in too

After reading the compilation of poems of this young poet in the book, *Let It Go: Voices from the Deep*, I would say, it is a very honest depiction of his thoughts and feelings, with no grain of artificiality. He has filled the words with emotions in exactly the shape and size they came, hence, every cell of his heart can be felt through the poems. But, those who look for the technical soundness of poetry might find flaws in the compiled content. Thus, I would like to conclude by saying that this young poet is like a seed which has a soft heart and a great promise to grow, and who would surely become a huge tree soon if watered well.

With all my good wishes and blessings, I congratulate Kinshuk for his first attempt at poetry.

Dr Mathura Dutt Pandey
26th July 2013

PREFACE

We live in a fast-paced world where we are so busy, that we forget to feel, enjoy, cry, and more importantly, love. When I say 'love', I mean not just romantic love, but love which defines us in various ways: togetherness, the love of nature, appreciating beauty, the love of God, being ourselves and sometimes the joy of finding ourselves. We all live in a beautiful world. Sometimes, we must pause, take a deep breath, and feel all the experiences with our senses.

As I thought more about it, I decided to give poetry a shot. My motivation was my maternal grandfather, Dr Mathura Dutt Pandey, who is an accomplished scholar of Sanskrit and Hindi Literature and had already written a lot of poems, for which he also received the President's Award. My mother used to recite his poems to me and I always enjoyed the sound of it, though I understood only a small part of what he wrote. Trying to follow in my grandfather's footsteps, I wrote my first English poem in 2009, which, to my surprise, came out better than I had expected. I got a lot of appreciation from my family and that was when my writing journey began.

As I attended a university which was next to the ocean, often I would go to the beach alone. Before I knew it, I fell in love with the ocean. A lot of my poems in this book have been inspired by what I felt and thought during my time at the ocean shore. Hence, I named the book *Let It Go: Voices from the Deep*.

This book is an attempt to give words to my observations, experiences and feelings as also to vent some of my frustrations. It is a bi-lingual compilation, in Hindi and English, comprising Ghazals and Nagme, poems, couplets and quatrains as well as songs. I have enjoyed putting together my thoughts and feelings and I hope you will enjoy reading it as much.

The Hindi verses and songs have been translated into English for the convenience of those who may not comprehend Hindi.

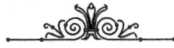

Ghazals & Nagme

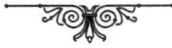

अटूट प्यार

प्यार में होते सितम, मैं हर सितम सह जाऊँगा
तुम भूलना जो चाहोगे, मैं अश्क बनकर आऊँगा।।

हुआ खत्म ना प्यार था फिर छोड़कर तुम क्यूँ गए
हाथ में कोई और चाहे, दिल में मैं ही आऊँगा।।

जा रही लहर-ए-मोहब्बत दिल का साहिल छोड़कर
जो तुम समन्दर में गए, मैं रेत बनकर आऊँगा।।

तन्हाई में याद तुमको जब हमारी आएगी
चाँद को तुम देखना मैं चाँदनी बन आऊँगा।।

≈

Unbreakable Love

Love is full of hardships but I'll bear them all
If you ever try to forget me, as your tears I would fall

Our love did not end, then why did you walk away?
Your hand might rest the world's, but your heart would be 'my' stay

The wave of love is leaving, but I'm glad I still see you
If you run in the sea, then, as sand I'd run in too

If lonely nights ever make you want to be on my side
As moonlight, I would come to you, you just don't need to hide

~

मोम सा दिल

मोम सा दिल हो ऐसे उसे गलाना हो
दिल जले मेरा रौशन कोई ज़माना हो।।

स्याह में चाँद ना दिखे तो चाँदनी भर दूँ
दर्द-ए-दिल को भी हँसने का इक बहाना हो।।

भँवरों की खातिर महकूँ मैं बनूँ फूल ऐसा
काँटे हो दिल में, महकी साँसों का नज़राना हो।।

लहर बन आऊँ हर बार फिसल जाऊँ पर मैं
यूँ ही तकदीर को शायद हमें मिलाना हो।।

हाल दुनिया का हो ऐसा छोड़कर जाऊँ जब मैं
दिल में आँधी हो, होंठों पे मुस्कुराना हो।।

∼

Heart of Wax

I wish of wax my heart be made
It lights the world when I do fade

If moon's not there, moonlight he spread
So hearts-in-pain can smile in bed

Though heart is thorned, for world he blooms
May he bleed fragrance for the lonely rooms

As a wave he steps, slips from the shore
Oh sand, Oh love, I'll try, once more!

When I die I wish, world would embrace
My emptiness with a smiling face

∼

फिर वो चल दिए

प्यार इस दिल में जगा के, फिर वो चल दिए
इक नई सुबह दिखा के, फिर वो चल दिए।।

था समा ना इश्क का, मौसम का जादू था
सर्द साँसों को बना के, फिर वो चल दिए।।

हम कमल थे वो भँवर, संग महके कुछ पल थे
इश्क का आँगन सजा के, फिर वो चल दिए।।

दिल के साहिल पर वो आए सीपियाँ बनकर
लहर की बातों में आ के, फिर वो चल दिए।।

इश्क के पँछी फँसे थे दिल के पिंजड़े में
उन परिंदों को उड़ा के, फिर वो चल दिए।।

स्याह में थी ज़िन्दगी पर साथ उनका था
सिसकियों की लौ जला के, फिर वो चल दिए।।

∼

And Then She Walked Away

She awoke my sleeping love, and then she walked away
Showed me the morning dove, and then she walked away

Love wasn't in the air, weather did spook a spell
Then chill came for a while, and then she walked away

I'm rose, she's butterfly, we had fun for a while
Fragrance spread in the sky, and then she walked away

My love, that shell, my love flowed in, onto my heart's shore
Sea played a cunning spy, and then she walked away

Stuck were the birds of love in the cage of my heart
She let those birdies fly, and then she walked away

My life was in the dark but still I had her love
She lit the lamp of cry, and then she walked away

≈

दामिनी–निर्भया

छूटने में दर्द तो क्यूँ छूटता ना दर्द है
फ़लक पे आफताब तो क्यूँ यह जहान सर्द है।।

सुनहरी चिड़िया देखकर दरिंदों ने उखाड़े पर
उड़ान जो ना दे सके,
हैवान है, नामर्द है।।

मेघ ने चुराया रंग तो
छुप गया था आसमान
बिजुर ने वार अब किया,
तड़प की ही यह नर्द है।।

आशाओं के मकान तो हर एक पल बनाए थे
हवस की एक आँधी से
हर इक मकान गर्द है।।

मातम भी विदाई है,
बस अश्क की नज़र अलग
इधर ना हौंसले बुलंद, इधर तो साँसें सर्द हैं।।

≈

Story of a Rape Victim

If pain comes in separation, separate pain from the bold
Sun I see in the horizon, then why world is so cold

The devils saw this golden bird, tore off her golden wings
Those creatures who can't help her fly,
are devils not human souls

When clouds (rapists) stole sky's colour (clothes),
the sky (victim) did hide its face
With lightning (rape) she is attacked today,
thunderous story is being told

Every second she laid some bricks to build her house of dreams
One storm of lust, that house came down,
each brick is soaked in mould

Her death or leaving (marriage) are the same
but for tears left behind
These tears are not full of hope, a loss is what they hold

~

संसार

अपनों को भी कैसे अपना कहूँ, दुश्मन अपने ही साए हैं
तुम अमन की दुनिया कहते हो, हम खूँ (खून) से नहाकर आए हैं।।

कहते हैं यहाँ सब मिलता है, सब इस पर ही रह जाता है
तुम दिल का मुकद्दर कहते हो, हम दिल दफ़नाकर आए हैं।।

जीवन के जहाजों पर अक्सर कुछ सैलाबों की रातें हैं
तुम जश्न-ए-समन्दर कहते हो,
हम लाशें बहा कर आए हैं।।

कल क्या होगा किसको ख़बर, यह आस से चलती दुनिया है
तुम उगता सूरज कहते हो,
हम कब्र सजाकर आए हैं।।

~

The World

My people aren't my own, my shadow is my enemy too
You said there's peace in the world, it's red I can't see blue

They say you get all you want here, it's all left in this place
You said here heart will fall in love, it fell for coffin screw

I'm a sailor on this ship of life, the ship does flood sometimes
You said I'd love this soothing jaunt,
my dead friends have loved it too

Tomorrow what would happen? The world just moves on hope
You said the sun would rise but,
My grave is calling? True

~

दिल मे क्यूँ

जानकर भी जानूँ ना मैं बेताबियाँ हैं दिल में क्यूँ
वादियाँ जब साथ मेरे वीरानियाँ हैं दिल में क्यूँ।।

कूक कोयल की ना सुनती, लहर भी ना बोलती है
शोर में जब सब फिज़ाएँ, खामोशियाँ हैं दिल में क्यूँ।।

रौशनी भी अब है रौशन, है सवेरा रात में भी
हर दिशा जब जगमगाए, स्याहियाँ हैं दिल में क्यूँ।।

प्यार से सकता निपट जो,
लड़-झगड़ के सब सुझाते
हर जिगर जब दम दिखाए,
कमज़ोरियाँ हैं दिल में क्यूँ।।

हर नशीली रात में सब
नाचते हैं यूँ चिपककर
जिस्म जब गर्मी बढ़ाए, तन्हाइयाँ हैं दिल में क्यूँ।।

~

Why

I know it but I still don't know why impatient is my heart
When lush nature is next to me, why barren is my heart?

I no more hear the nightingale, even the waves are silent
When there is noise all around, why quiet is my heart?

Light I can see everywhere, it's day even at night
When every place is so well-lit, why blackened is my heart?

Most of the problems just need love,
but they're all ready to fight
When every person feels so strong,
why weakness fills their heart?

They grind, they dance, hug every chance,
when night is full of booze
When body feels the body warmth, why lonely is their heart?

~

बेवफ़ाई

और की बाहों में थे वो, देखा यह नज़ारा है
हम सोचते रहे की उनको इन्तज़ार हमारा है।।

नदिया भी चहकी थी कि सागर से मिलेगी
नादान को मालूम ना कि हर समन्दर खारा है।।

इक दिल ही था हमारा रहा साथ जो हमेशा
इश्क के जुए में आज टूटा दिल भी हारा है।।

सोचा जलती किरणों ने कि तारों सी ठंडक मिले
समझाया तब किताब ने सूरज भी इक सितारा है।।

है अब ना कोई दिलबरा, पर तन्हा हम नहीं हैं
इस इश्क के जहान में ग़म ही इक सहारा है।।

~

Cheating

I saw her dance with someone else, in his arms she did halt
I thought she's waited all this while, I guess it's just my fault

The river jumped to see the sea, 'that water would be pure'
But little did she know that sea is full of minerals, salt

My heart has been my greatest friend, it's never left my side
I gambled even him in love, it has all been my fault

The solar rays once saw the stars, wished to be cool like them
The book explained to one and all, star even sun is called

Today though no one loves me through, but still I'm not alone
Love has a lonely world in which sorrow does give a call

~

प्यार ना मिला

सब मिला इक जीने का आधार ना मिला
इस जहान में बस तुम्हारा प्यार ना मिला।।

इश्क में जाती है जानें, लोग मरते हैं
ज़िन्दगी को मौत का दरबार ना मिला।।

घूम आया हूँ मैं सारे देश दुनिया के
सब मिला इक प्यार का संसार ना मिला।।

देख तुमको जाने ना क्यूँ आँख रोती है
हर नज़र को शायद एतबार ना मिला।।

छूटता है वो जो प्यार से बँधा कभी
दिल तलब को छूटने का भार ना मिला।।

~

Couldn't Find Love

I found everything, but couldn't find a living way
They say love is all I need, but you were gone for the day

They say people fall in love, they say people die in love
I have been unlucky enough, even death did not obey

I've travelled every place, every country of this world
I've lived in every town, but in love I could not stay

I don't know why I cry every time I see your face
I guess my lonely eye, still hears the words you say

Broken is that man who has been truly loved some time
My heart is broken too, for, not been broken for a day

~

जुदाई

इश्क वो करते थे हमसे वो ज़माना ढह गया
नयनों से निकली नदी में दिल हमारा बह गया।।

धुन जो छेड़ी तूने उस पल हर फिज़ा महकाई थी
वादियाँ दिल की में अब बस नग्मों का रस रह गया।।

मेघ के कण-कण ने हम पर प्यार ही बरसाया था
दाग़ शोलों का बदन पर आज सावन दे गया।।

मौत से डरता था मैं तुझे छोड़ना मुमकिन नहीं
चन्द पलों की याद से यह ज़िंदगी मैं सह गया।।

❧

Separation

That season is long gone when she used to love me
I've drowned in my tears, my soul's left free

Where can I find those days, when you sang your fragrance out
Today I know the words, but that heart I cannot see

Every cell of cloud used to shower love on us
Even those raindrops now drop burning coal on me

Death used to scare me because I could not leave you
Your memories are just left, don't take them, let them be

≈

मिटा नहीं यह प्यार है

दूरियों के आने से मिटा नहीं यह प्यार है
हाथ छूट जाने से मिटा नहीं यह प्यार है।।

खत जला दिए जला दी प्यार की निशानियाँ
यादों को जलाने से मिटा नहीं यह प्यार है।।

तू है शायद और की, हूँ मैं भी शायद और का
ये गुत्थियाँ सुलझाने से मिटा नहीं यह प्यार है।।

नयनों से बरस रही है
हाल-ए-दिल की इक ग़ज़ल
यह शायरी छुपाने से मिटा नहीं यह प्यार है।।

होंठ बोलते हैं वो जो दिल मे बात है नहीं
सच का दिल दुखाने से
मिटा नहीं यह प्यार है।।

≈

Love Doesn't End There

Distances do come, but love doesn't end there
Hands are left by some, but love doesn't end there

I put your letters in the fire, and everything of you
I did not leave a single crump, but love doesn't end there

Was I even made for her, was she too made for me?
Even if I can solve this sum, but love doesn't end there

My empty eyes have rained poems,
straight from my wounded heart
All of them? No I didn't hum, but love doesn't end there

Your lips convey a message that your heart don't want to say
You hurt the truth, that act was dumb,
but love doesn't end there

~

इक आख़िरी बार

नज़रें नहीं तो यादों को देदे पनाह, इक आख़िरी बार
ज़ुल्मत-ए-ख़ुमार में फिर होने दे फ़ना, इक आख़िरी बार।।

चाँदनी रात है, तेरे हुस्न में खोने दे मुझे
शब्नम-ए-हसरत आज तू कर न मना, इक आख़िरी बार।।

तन्हा मंज़र है, तेरे साथ की गुज़ारिश हूँ करता
रंजिश-ए-शाम की गीली याद बना, इक आख़िरी बार।।

दिल के खण्डहर में दीप तू रख जा बिन लौ के चाहे
तेरे आने से ही गुमनाम हो अँधकार घना, इक आख़िरी बार।।

~

One Last Time

If not to my self, just hug my thought, one last time
Then let me drown in that love you brought, one last time

It's a moonlit night, let me lose myself in your beauty today
That time is here please don't say not, one last time

My surroundings feel so lonely, I yearn for your company
Just come, I'll give you all I've got, one last time

Keep a lamp in my heart's dungeon, maybe that has no wick
Your presence only will light the rot, one last time

~

जानूँ नहीं

ज़हर या अमृत पिया, ये तो मैं जानूँ नहीं
किस नज़र को घर दिया, ये तो मैं जानूँ नहीं।।

अप्सराएँ हर तरफ, मैं प्यार का था बादशाह
पर इश्क क्या मैंने किया, ये तो मैं जानूँ नहीं।।

आया तेरे शहर में दिल अपने का पैग़ाम ले
जान-ए-दिल किसको दिया, ये तो मैं जानूँ नहीं।।

जल चुका था प्यार में इज़हार जो ना कर सका
होंठों को फिर क्यूँ सिया, ये तो मैं जानूँ नहीं।।

सैलाब-ए-हुस्न में फँसा जाल-ए-नज़र बस इक उम्मीद
किसकी पलकों पर जिया, ये तो मैं जानूँ नहीं।।

रात मय में धुत करी
नशा इश्क का जब सो गया
किस नशे ने दम लिया, ये तो मैं जानूँ नहीं।।

≈

I Don't Know

Poison or nectar did I drink, I don't know
Whose love could reach my heart's brink, I don't know

Fairies were at every place, I was the king of love
But did in love I ever sink, I don't know

I reached your city with a text, a message of my heart
To which heart was that message linked, I don't know

I was already burnt as I could not express my love then
Why my lips, still, could not sing, I don't know

Flood of beauty, I was stuck, a love-sight net could save
In whose eyelashes did I blink, I don't know

I boozed the night when love was boozed,
the booze was boozing too
Which booze pushed me off the brink, I don't know

~

क्या करूँ

झुकती पलकों ने जो कहा उस बात का मैं क्या करूँ
महताब भी अब ना रहा, इस रात का मैं क्या करूँ।।

मेरे प्यार को परदा किया नज़र-ए-जहाँ को छोड़कर
फिर आँसू में तू क्यूँ बहा, इस साथ का मैं क्या करूँ।।

हाथों में तेरा हाथ ले चाहूँ मैं तुझमें डूबना
जो हाथ तेरा ना मिले, इस हाथ का मैं क्या करूँ।।

दुनिया से हारूँ ग़म नहीं एहसास गर तेरा रहे
मैं आज हारी तुझसे भी, इस मात का मैं क्या करूँ।।

What Should I Do

What your dropping lash said, words, what should I do with it
The moon too now has set, night, what should I do with it

You locked my love all alone, and left the world of my eyes
Came back in tears, company, what should I do with it

Hand in hand I'd walk with you, I want to drown in you
Today you left my hand, my hand, what should I do with it

I don't care if I lose the world, if you are there with me
Today I even lost you, loss, what should I do with it

~

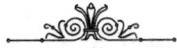

Hindi Poetry

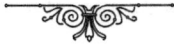

सागर तट पर

समुद्र है, ज़मीन भी है,
हर साँस तो थमी भी है
सन्नाटे के संगीत की,
मुस्कान में नमी भी है
समुद्र है, ज़मीन भी है।।

अठखेलियों के गीत में, भावनाओं का स्वर गूँजता
ब्रह्मांड भी क्षितिजांत तक, कुछ प्यार के पल ढूँढता
मोती से आँखें है सजी, और दिल मे कुछ कमी भी है
समुद्र है, ज़मीन भी है।।

हर एक झोंका प्यार से, इस दिल का दर्द पूछता
आवाज़ देता मैं उसे, वो साथ मेरे रूँधता
इन झोंकों के एहसास में, तन्हाई की गमी भी है
समुद्र है, ज़मीन भी है, हर साँस तो थमी भी है।।

❧

On the Ocean Shore

Ocean I see, I see the shore
Seeing it, a bit my breath has slowed
There's a silent music in the waves
Through my eyes a story is told
Ocean I see, I see the shore

Wave's echoing hurt in every song
For love, sky too seems to have craved
My eyes are dropping priceless pearls
A lonely road, my heart has paved

I shouted at the ocean song
A spell of breeze calmed me again
Even that soothing breeze that came
Seemed to be drinking love of pain

Ocean I see, I see the shore
Seeing it, a bit my breath has slowed
There's a silent music in the waves
Through my eyes a story is told

~

बगिया, नदिया

मेरी यह बगिया ऐसी है, मेरी यह नदिया ऐसी है
कई जीवों की खाद है इसमें,
कई नहरें आबाद है इसमें
असली माटी की सूँघ कहाँ पर,
अपने कँकर की गूँज कहाँ पर
मिश्रण की सुविधा ऐसी या, मिश्रण की दुविधा ऐसी है
मेरी यह बगिया ऐसी है, मेरी यह नदिया ऐसी है।।

सूखी भू भी हँसी वहाँ जहाँ अलि सारे अब झूम रहे हैं
इन्द्रधनुष के सातों घोड़े बागान में ही घूम रहे हैं
बचपन के वो खेल कहाँ पर, मासूमियत की वो बेल कहाँ पर
आकर्षण की सुविधा ऐसी या, आकर्षण की दुविधा ऐसी है
मेरी यह बगिया ऐसी है, मेरी यह नदिया ऐसी है।।

कई नदों का मेल यह ऐसा, स्वर्ग-लोक का अमृत लगता
जन्म-मरण की डोर बाँधकर, मग समस्त को पावन करता
हिमनद के वो श्वास कहाँ पर, हिमगिरी का एहसास कहाँ पर
परिवर्तन की सुविधा ऐसी या, परिवर्तन की दुविधा ऐसी है
मेरी यह बगिया ऐसी है, मेरी यह नदिया ऐसी है।।

My Garden, My River

That is how my garden is, that is how my river is
Manure is mixed to grow the tea
A lot of rivers merge in me
But now 'my' soil I cannot smell
Where is 'my' drop? Oh! What the hell
Is mixture boon or mixture bane?
That is what my garden asks, that is what my river asks

Dry mud laughed where butterflies fly
The flowers have bloomed, rainbow ain't shy
But now I see no childhood game
No water-ice, no teaming blame
Is pretty boon or pretty bane?
That is what my garden asks, that is what my river asks

Yes, I flow the holy water
All worship me; the son, the daughter
But I don't see my glacial snow
No icy-breath, just crowded flow
Is change a boon or change a bane?
That is what my garden asks, that is what my river asks

≈

आबादगी

खुशबुओं को सूँघ के जो फूल तोड़ें हम
भँवरों की जान के कातिल नहीं हैं कम
पुष्प की पाखों पर सुख की नींद जब सोए
सोच भी पाए नहीं क्या फूल थे रोए
दर्द-ए-आँसू दे खुशी नहीं जीत है वो हार
लेना ही है दर्द लो आबाद हो संसार।।

लहरों को देखो गौर से सागर से जब मिलती
कुछ ये ले जाती हैं कुछ सागर को हैं देती
आसमाँ भी पानी को रंग अपना है देता
नर जान देना भूलकर अब जान ही लेता
इन्सानियत का खून कर मिलता नहीं है प्यार
लेना ही है दर्द लो आबाद हो संसार।।

पेड़ों को देखो यह खगों को रहने की जगह देते
प्यार की सीमा न बाँधे एक जुट रहते
बाँटकर धरती भला क्या खुश रहेंगे हम
दिल के टुकड़े कर के देख यह तोड़ देगा दम
मनुज की है जीत तब जब दिल पर हो ना वार
लेना ही है दर्द लो आबाद हो संसार।।

Prosperity

We pluck the flowers that do smell good
Are we less monsters for the bees?
We love romance on petals of rose
Did rose feel pain? What about the trees?
It ain't no love in that blood-stained room
Try take their tears, the world will bloom

Notice the waves when they meet the shore
They take some with, they give some more
The sky too gives its colour to the sea
We need to give life, instead we take three
We can't find love, if humans we doom
Try take their tears, the world will bloom

Learn from the trees, they give birds a home
They make no borders, no Sparta no Rome
Will we ever be happy, by cutting into states
Cut open your heart, know what'll happen with hate
Let's change this world, the world full of gloom
Try take their tears, the world will bloom

∽

मोहब्बत

होंठों पर हैं बोल कई पर कहने से मन डरता है
आँखों में हैं शोक नहीं फिर दिल क्यूँ पल-पल भरता है
नशा-ए-इश्क यह ऐसा है हर माही जन्नत पाता है
मोहब्बत के इस सागर में हर राही डूब के जाता है।।

हँसते भी आँसू बहते हैं,
रोने में भी अब ग़म नहीं
दिल में ना हो वो तो लगता, जीवन है बस हम नहीं
आँधी का भी रुख बदलता,
मस्ताना वो कहलाता है
मोहब्बत के इस सागर में हर राही डूब के जाता है।।

सपनो मे रहनेवालों को सोने मे भी अब चैन नहीं
ग़ालिब की खुशबू जिस दर पर,
आँखें नज़रों की हैं वहीं
दुनिया कहती है इसको इश्क, सबको जादू यह भाता है
मोहब्बत के इस सागर में हर राही डूब के जाता है।।

~

Love

A lot of words rest on the lips that the heart is scared to say
There is no sorrow in my eyes, then why is heart heavy all day
Love is such that everyone feels like the heaven's dove
At some point you would take a plunge in this ocean of love

Sometimes tears flow in a happy state,
some sadness skips the cry
Her presence does decorate the world, her absence makes it dry
That which can change the flow of storms,
such is this heaven's dove
At some point you would take a plunge in this ocean of love

People who love to stay in dreams, now find it hard to sleep
Their eyes keep searching for her voice,
her fragrance does run deep
Everyone loves this magic city, where lives the heaven's dove
At some point you would take a plunge in this ocean of love

~

क्या दुनिया, क्या जन्नत

सदियों बाद खोली हैं आँखें, जाना पहचाना कुछ नहीं
चल चुका हूँ मील कई, रास्ते दिखते कई
देख सकता हूँ सभी कुछ, कैसी दिखती है ज़मीन
खूबसूरत हर कहीं, यह खूबसूरत हर कहीं।।

सूर्य की पहली किरण से, हर कली चुँधिया रही
लाल–पीली पत्तियाँ भी मग्न बहती जा रहीं
हर नज़ारा ऐसा है, होंठों को शब्दों की कमी
आँखों की जन्नत यही है, आँखों की जन्नत यही।।

पर दिल के दिल का क्या हुआ? उस प्रेम रस का क्या हुआ?
आँगन वह उजड़ा रह गया, दीप बिन जले ही बह गया
तब दिखता था ना यह समां, धुंधला सा लगता था जहाँ
पर दिल का आँगन था भरा, मन का भंवर भी था जवाँ
दिल उस समय भी खोया था, दिल इस समय भी खोया है
दोनो में फ़र्क बस इतना है, दिल बेज़ुबान अब रोया है
उड़ चुका हूँ दूर मैं, पर दिल न मेरा उड़ सका
रहता हूँ जन्नत में अब, पर दुनिया मेरी उस जगह
मझधार में हूँ मैं खड़ा, मुझे दोनो मिल सकता नहीं
फिर देखूँ आँखें मूँदकर, जन्नत यहीं दिल भी यहीं ।।।

What's World, What's Heaven

I'm conscious after so long, nothing now seems familiar
I've walked a million miles, I see a million ways
I can see everything now, through nights and the days
It's beautiful everywhere, it's indeed beautiful everywhere

With the first ray of the sun, each bud smiles with joy
Red, yellow leaves too float merrily in the breeze
The spectacle is so pretty, my lips fumble for words
A paradise I see, my eyes feel at ease

But what really happened to the heart of my heart?
What really happened to that nectar of love?
Was that garden ever made? Nope
Did the heat get some shade? Nope
Agreed, it wasn't this pretty that time
Agreed, the world was hazy
At least there were smiles off and on
At least I wasn't crazy
My heart then felt the burn, but heart now seems to fry
Eyes dropped a tear then, now drops the silent cry
I've flown a place too far, my heart couldn't fly with me
This heaven I don't need, if my heart I cannot see
Can both be there with me? Well, life shows me a No
Again I close my eyes, both are part of the show

ज़िंदगी की राह

ज़िंदगी की राह मे कहीं रात है,
दिन है कहीं
लक्ष्य धुंधला है यहाँ, हर राह भी दिखती नहीं
दिल में तूफान उठ रहे, झंझा में तू है भीगता
कल कल में ही रहता तू, क्यूँ आज से ना सीखता
फिक्र के अंधकार में तू
सूर्य को ना पाएगा
राही तू आगे बढ़ता जा,
पथ खुद-ब-खुद बन जाएगा ।।

सोचता क्यूँ हर पहर तू
बचा सके पूँजी जमा
इक बात तू यह जान ले सुख से बड़ा ना कुछ यहाँ
खुद का सभी यहाँ सोचते, फ़कीरों की तू बात कर
किसी और को चलना सिखा, किसी और की झोली तू भर
इन तारों के आँचल तले फिर प्यार ही तू पाएगा
राही तू आगे बढ़ता जा,
पथ खुद-ब-खुद बन जाएगा ।।

Road of Life

The roads of life don't stay the same,
there's day and there is night
The milestones are hazy too, it's hard to take a flight
There'd be some storms of aspirations roaring in your heart
History, mystery, forget it now, today is where you start
The storm might try to stop you but winds aren't there to stay
Just keep walking with all your faith,
the road will show the way

Why do you think what you have earned,
someone is going to steal?
You're smile is the 'most precious' here, there is no better deal
All here care for their very self, you care for lonely souls
Teach someone to drop a smile, help someone fill their bowls
You give a bit, you'd get a lot, with love the world will pay
Just keep walking with all your faith,
the road will show the way

~

दबंग

नीले अम्बर की ढाल हूँ मैं
तूफानों का भी काल हूँ मैं
गुमनाम गुफा से डरता जो
उस राही की मशाल हूँ मैं
ना देव ना महापुरुष मैं
ना मैं कोई मसीहा हूँ
लहू माँस का पुतला हूँ मैं
साँसों पर ही जीता हूँ
पर मन में है जुनून ऐसा
हर गूँगे की आवाज़ हूँ मैं
तुम दिल में आग लगा देखो फिर
तुमसा ही जाँबाज़ हूँ मैं।।

❦

The Saviour

I am the armour of the sky
Storm will be dead because I am here
The one who's scared to walk the dark
I am his lamp to shed his fear
I'm neither God nor superman
His messenger? Well, no I am not
I too am made of flesh and blood
I too can smell the country rot
But I've a heart with passion filled
A passion that is true
Just burn with passion in your heart
Then I am just like you

≈

डरता हूँ मैं

ज़िन्दगी नहीं
दिल टूट जाने से
डरता हूँ मैं।।

बदन नहीं
दिल जल जाने से
डरता हूँ मैं।।

माना तन है
पर इश्क़ है मेरा
बेजान नहीं।।

तन को देख
तेरे छोड़ जाने से
डरता हूँ मैं।।

~

I am Scared

Not of death
From broken heart
Yes, I am scared

Not burnt body
From burnt heart
Yes, I am scared

Yes, I'm weak
But my love is
Stronger than else's

Seeing my body
You would leave
Yes, I am scared

~

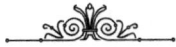

English Poetry

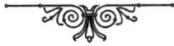

Let it Go

Hand in hand I walked
On the golden sand
With sea waves whistling to me
Look at my beauty
My clear water, my blue lagoon
Hold me close in your palms
Just as the love you share
With chill on my face, with warmth in my heart
I felt the ocean calling
Through my feet, through my soul
I lifted a few majestic drops
Of beauty, of grace, of the ocean
And held the love of nature in my palm with all I had
As if it was all I had
I opened my palm, I lost some love
I made a fist, still lost some love
I did not care of the ocean left
Falling love just made me low
Harder I tried, more I cried
And then I had to let it go

Love left me
From my palm, then from my life
My heart felt the slit

As it drowned again in those majestic drops
Not from the ocean, but from my eyes this time
I held that tear
As long as I could, as hard as I could
The tear that had my world in it
Every feeling, every emotion, every memory
The tear that meant the world to me
I held it. Not felt it, not lived it
Just held it
My heart suffocated, my eyes blinded
But still I didn't let it flow
I thought I would never say goodbye
But then I had to let it go

All my life I was told
Strength is what defines a man
Emotional, Mental, Physical
Not either but and
Holding on was for the strong
That made us strong
But then I learnt the greatest truth
Life made sure I should know
The strongest have a little more
They've learnt to let it go

∾

Alice in Wonderland

I close my eyes
I see a light amidst the darkness
A light that surrounds you
It's like a lighted painting on a black background
Maybe a 3D painting with a bulb inside
Or maybe it's just your glow: I don't know
It's so well done that I can see it all
Every single detail
What I see is so beautiful
Red dress with red cheeks, open hair, confused looks,
pretty smile
Oh! I can go on for days together
You look like a princess, a princess from fairytales
It's so heart-warming
I want to reach you, hold you, hug you, till the end of time
But you're standing too far
I walk towards you but I get no closer
I feel like on a treadmill: I can't move forward
You're so close yet so far
I'm trying so hard: Why don't you come closer?
Wait! Where did you just go? I can't see you anymore
I guess my eyes just opened
What I see now is reality: a reality I don't want to be in
These lights blind me

The sounds feel like poking needles
I want to close my eyes. I do
And I'm back. It's so peaceful in here
I see you're still standing there
I still can't reach you but it's okay
At least I can see you, as long as I want
I'm so glad to be back
To this land so quiet, where no sound hurts me
To this land not so bright, where only you I see
To this land of my dreams, the one that I paint
But not alone: with my Alice in Wonderland!

~

Desire

In all this loneliness, I close my eyes
And reach the fairy land
The waves playing the music
The breeze is whispering to me
'Treasure this moment for there'd be nothing in the world
That'd make you feel better than this.
That, at the same time
Would make you laugh and cry
Would make you live and die
Would make you strong and weak
Would give you all you seek'

I see light in the darkness
I feel warmth in the chill
Am I going crazy? Am I getting sick?
Or is the sea breeze just playing a trick?

I look to my right and see you sitting next to me
Looking at the stars and listening to the sea
Now I know exactly what is happening to me
The light is your glow; the warmth is your touch
The stars too look pretty. As you? Not so much
I take a closer look at your beautiful face
At those eyes that reflect a million emotions, so honest and pure

At that smile that takes me to a different world
The world I call paradise
At that lock of hair that plays on your face in the breeze
Every passing second feels like a dream
A dream I wish I could live in, as long I would be
A dream where I could walk with you, near the sea
A dream where I don't have to miss you ever again
You're all I need to end this pain

~

Enlightenment

You look left, you look right
There is no land you can find
All you see is the ocean water
Quiet waves, some ripples. And life? Maybe
Amidst the divinity of Mother Nature
Dawning sky; red, orange, some blue, some black
Soothing breeze, chilly enough to make you feel
The feeling of hope. A new day is being born
You feel the stillness, of the breeze, of the boat, time, of life
It's more like a dream, a dream so pure, so real
That you're left with no option, but to drop a tear
Your eyes can't hold it, neither your heart, nor your soul
Because this world you see is where you always wanted to be
Because this world you embrace is the only place
Where you can be who you are, how you are
No faces, no obligations, nothing. Just one truth
A truth you forgot long time back,
Of who you are, how you are
Live the moment, embrace it
Let yourself loose
Flow in the serenity: the serenity where you will find you
The cage is gone, the shackles broken
Freedom is what you smell
Enlightenment!

Outlook

Life is a word that can be plain or can be very deep
You look at it with positive eyes and pleasure you will reap
You deem its fun it will be so you don't even have to try
You start to whine about it then it'll surely make you cry

It gives you joy and fun, it sings the merry song
Though it can be harsh sometimes, it's just to make you strong
It gives you these ups and downs to fill this trip with qualm
This way it separates optimists
while others get stuck in a swamp

People who cross this swampy land
are successes of the human race
Others drown to the swampy bed without leaving a trace
They struggle and cry; get depressed and whine about this trip
Who is to blame for what they're in?
They were the captain of their ship

The best thing about this trip is that
to turn it is never too late
The time you generate positive thoughts
it'll be your greatest mate
The day we're born we captain this ship;
no one escapes this jaunt

It's you who'd decide what you want from life,
a friend or a ghost that'd haunt

~

I—The God

I gave them life and air to breathe
I gave them whatever their heart could need
I made Mother Nature, so they could play for pleasure
I gave them a soul, which I asked them to treasure

They reached the new world and named it 'Earth'
A place of abundance, where there was no dearth
They enjoyed everything from the rains to the sea
They were happy playing around the flowers and the tree

In this happy place, no one was able to read
The evil greedy thoughts that had started to breed
'We would rule the world' was all they said
For this they started colouring my best creation red

They shot some on their head; they stabbed some in their heart
They smiled when people suffered; they tore families apart
They raided hotels, blew it up with grenade
They've brought the sunny earth under a deathly shade

They've forgotten the promise they made before they went
They are the main reason for earth to have a dent
Now if they want to fight, they have to fight with me
Or they have to live in peace, like it was meant to be.

Is it Destiny?

Whenever you open the newspaper the headline always says
Crimes all over the world are increasing now-a-days
They kill people for a few bucks,
they follow their animal instinct
If the rate goes on like this,
soon human race would be extinct

People think they're dodgy creatures
because they break all the laws
Though no one dares to think deep enough
to reach the root cause
I was forced to think this way when I read about a boy
Who at the age of eight made weapons his toy

It wasn't that he was poor enough to buy a toy joker
His family was slaughtered mercilessly
when caught in the trap of a broker
The boy approached the police for help
but they refused him the same
He took the criminal route and he wasn't to be blamed

He found the broker in a month and killed him with his knife
The same police that refused him help was now after his life
He thought of leaving this business but there was no return

The art of evading the police was
the first thing that he learnt

Stations and airports were informed;
entry to his house was closed
He had no food, no place to stay, yet he remained composed
He saw the police laying a trap
when he went to get some water
To be safe from the cops,
he kidnapped the commissioner's daughter

The innocent girl was kidnapped at one
when no one was at home
He took her to a secret room behind the palace dome
He called up the commissioner from a booth
and asked a path to run
Said if he refused to help, then his girl wouldn't see the sun

The officer had a plan in mind,
to the boy the commissioner lied
The boy soon found out his intent and so the poor girl died
His hideouts were out by then as his friend was highly paid
The boy was shot right on his head and in nature's lap he
laid

The media showed him encountered;
his death was not a myth
The inspector who shot the dangerous boy

was given a laurel wreath
The crimes he did were not his choice,
circumstances made him do
Criminals are human after all,
just like me and you

~

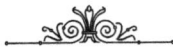

Couplets & Quatrains

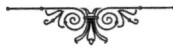

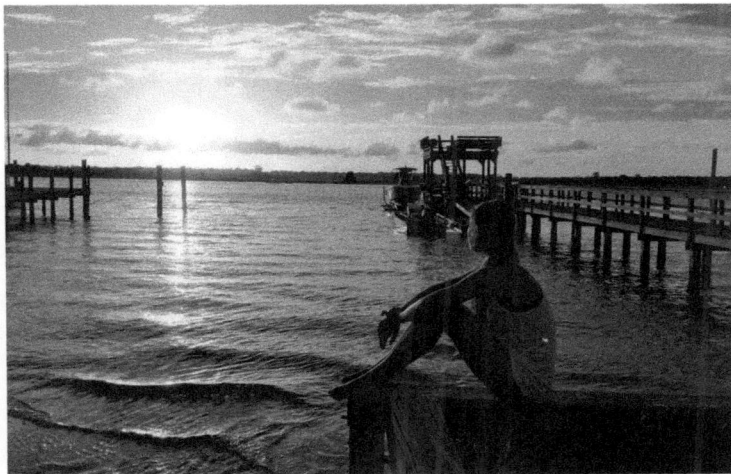

Photograph by Angie Sakely

I see the dawn diamond: yellow, orange and brown
If land is a princess, the sky is the crown
I see the waves dancing to the tune of the breeze
In the world I live, I've never felt this ease
I've heard people say life is full of surprise
I guess then on earth, I just witnessed paradise

~

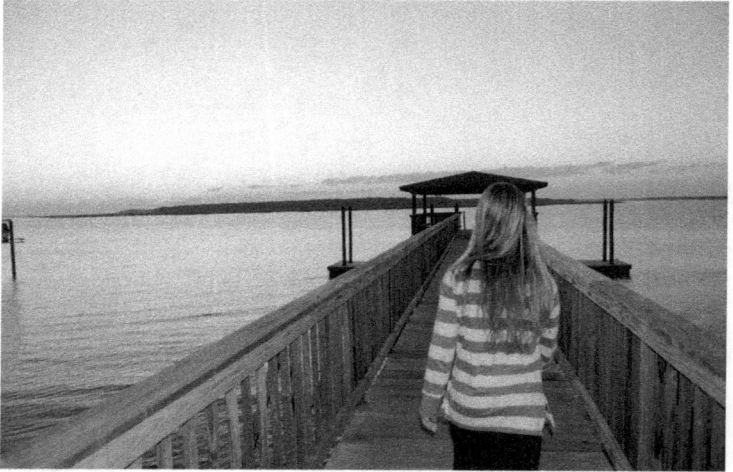

Photograph by Kelly Cameron

The dancing waves, the playful tides
The singing breeze, is what I show
But there's a deeper world within
With secrets you would never know

∾

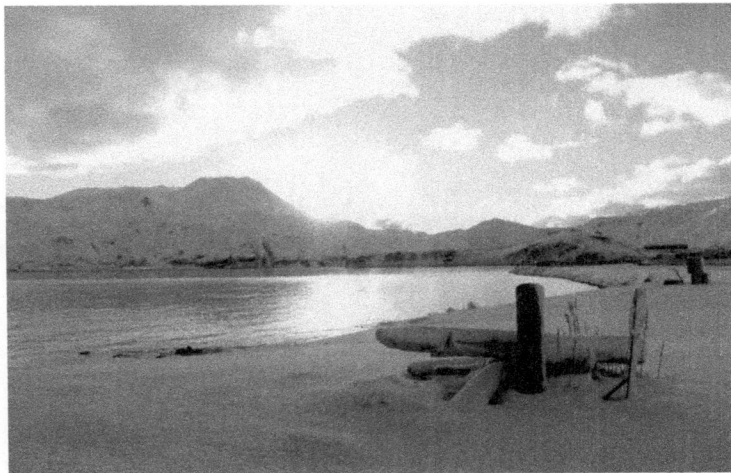

Photograph by Samantha Ehnert

Tears today are smiles tomorrow
Both are yours, no one can borrow
Too much heat will make you sick
There's some chill in every sorrow

∾

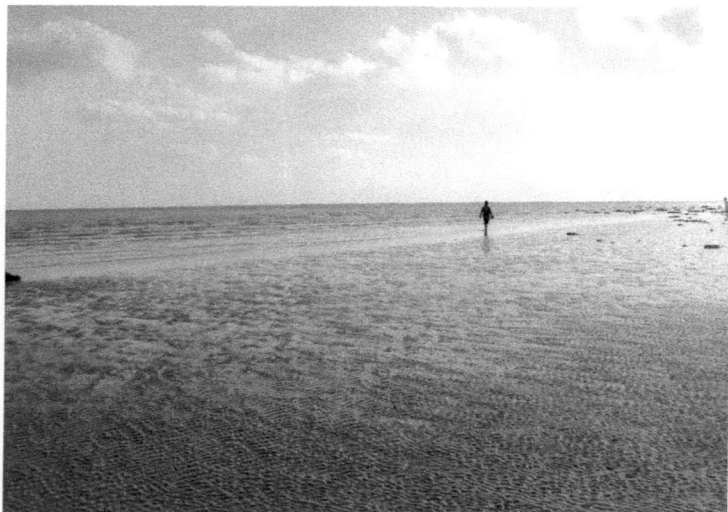

Photograph by Garima Sharma

Alone I walk in this place so calm
No pain in the world I see
Waves at my feet, sands on my palm
At last I'm the living me

∾

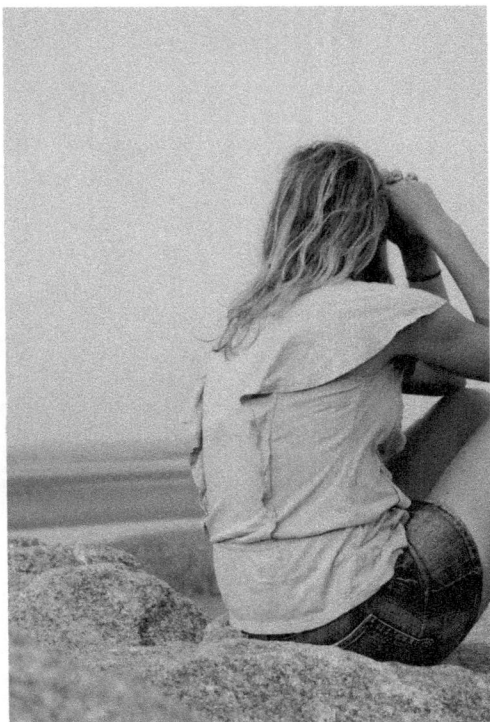

Photograph by Kelly Cameron

I did my best—got called a thief
Touched highest sky—pushed in a reef
Sun gives the light, moon takes the prize
There'll be a dawn, don't lose belief

~

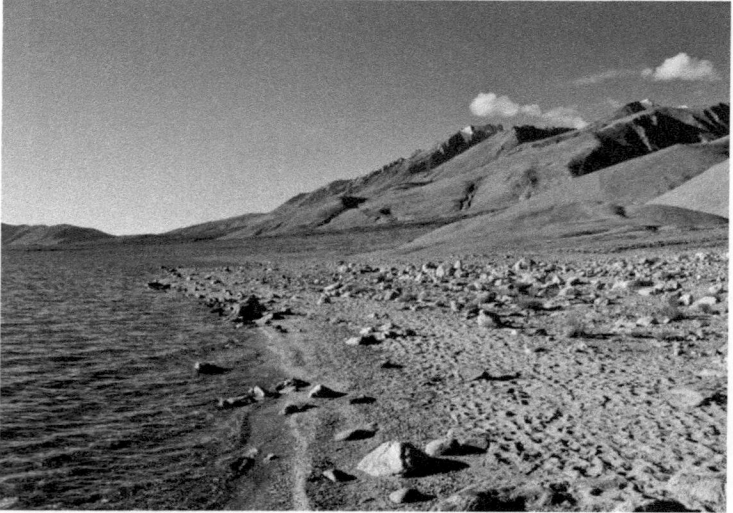

Photograph by Varad Tripathi

The world may say I'm made of stone
But I try to love the sky
I also hug the lonely sea
I soothe a lonely eye
Life for me is happiness
In others that I see
I give some smiles to all I can
I get my own for free

~

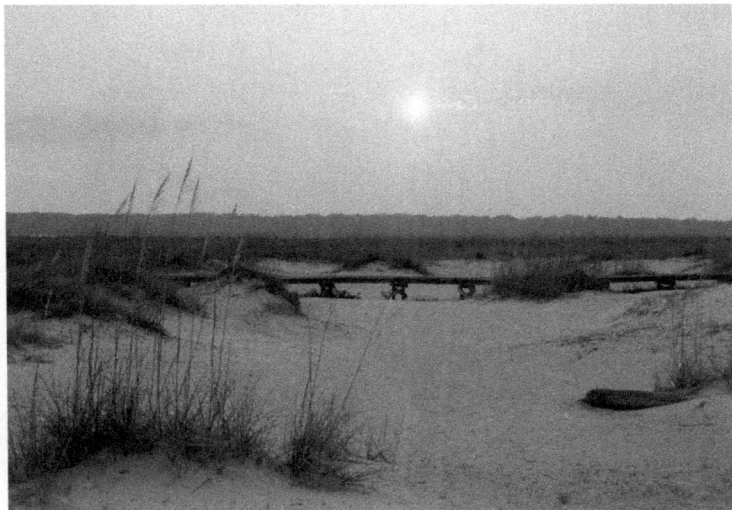

Photograph by Kelly Cameron

Life hits dusk, life hits dawn
People you love are one day gone
The tree ain't sad when nature acts
A flower is dead but a fruit is born
Butterflies won't live, if caterpillars don't die
When a soul leaves skin, it's not a goodbye
It's a change of gear from the one that's torn
When death means life, why do people mourn?

~

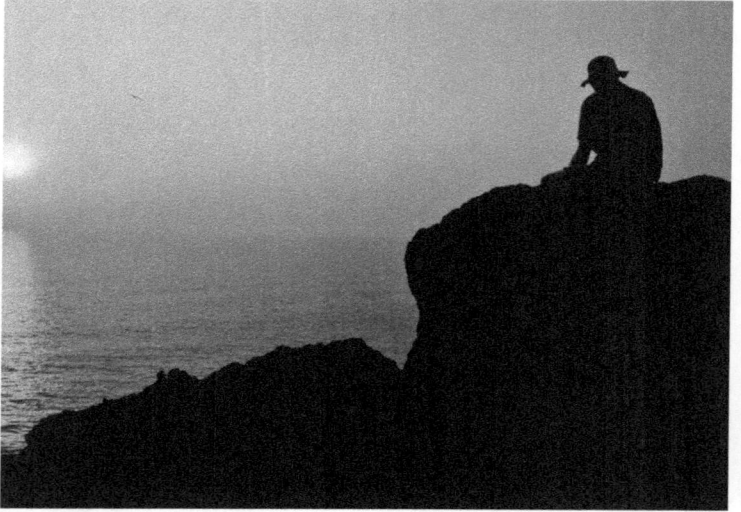

Photograph by Varad Tripathi

तेरी बेरहम नज़रों को दिल से लगा रखूँगा
सुना है यहाँ पत्थर में भी ख़ुदा होता है।।

Even your stone-like love I'll keep close to my heart
I've heard here God resides even in stone

~

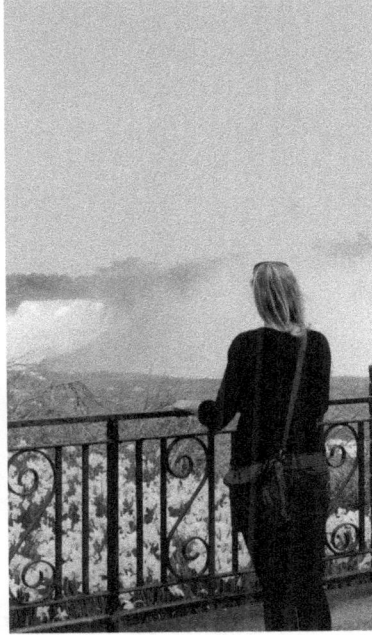

Photograph by Kelly Cameron

पैसे के नयन कई, मैं ढूँढूँ प्यार की नज़र
साँस लेते कई दिखे, ज़िंदगी देखूँ इधर।।

Money gets a lot of eyes, my eyes search a loving stare
I've seen a lot of those who breathe, At last, life I can see here

~

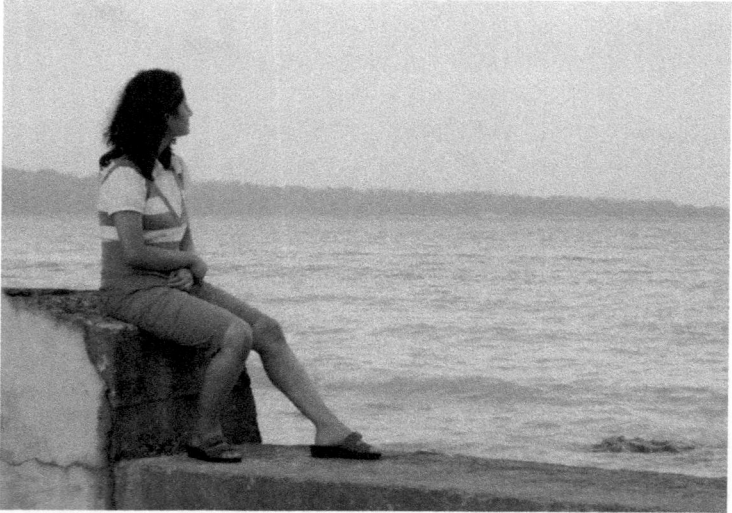

Photograph by Kinshuk Sharma

लहर-ए-मोहब्बत देखती हूँ आज तन्हा इस कदर
कि साथ साँसें भी जो छोड़ें अब फ़रक पड़ता नहीं।।

I see the waves of love today, my heart still feels so shattered
Even if breath leaves me today, how does it even matter

~

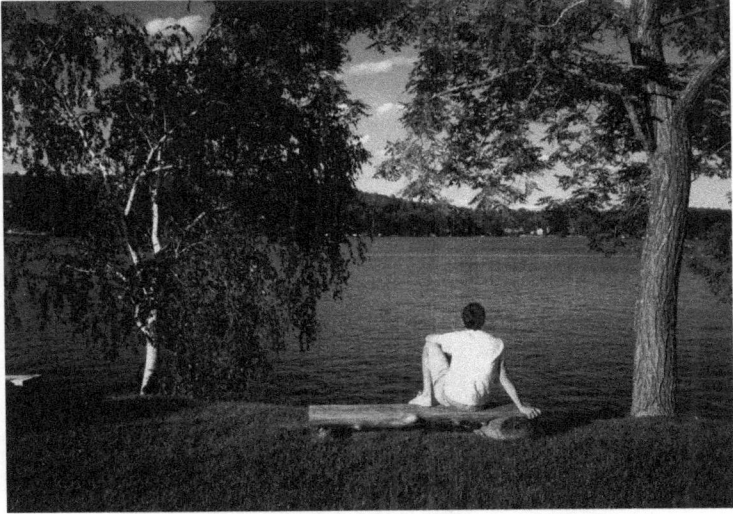

Photograph by Alex Wetherell and Liana McHugh

छुआ इन हवाओं ने आज चेहरे को इस क़दर
कि फिर उनकी ज़ुल्फ़ों की मुझे याद आ गई।।

The breeze touched my face today in such a way
That memories of her flowing hair hugged me again

~

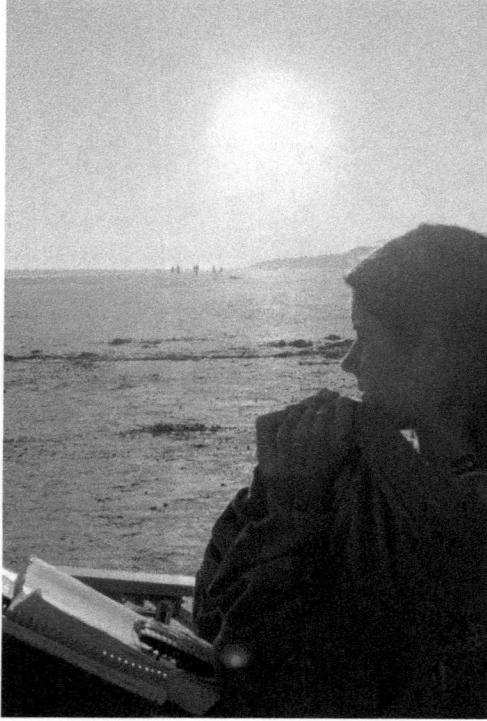

Photograph by Kelly Cameron

छोड़ा उसने नाम जिसका साहिल-ए-दिल पर लिखा था
आँसुओं की बारिश मे वो नाम आज डुबा रही हूँ।।

He left whose name I had written on the shore of my heart
Today I am drowning that name in the rain of my tears

~

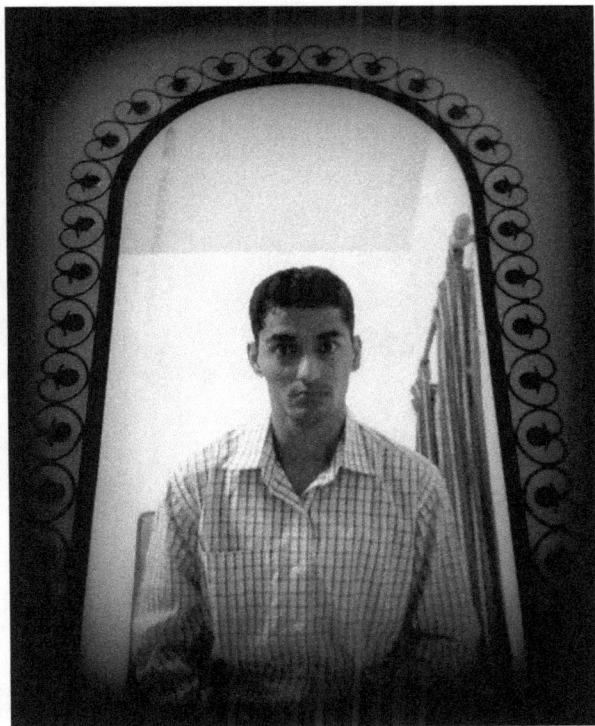

Photograph by Kinshuk Sharma

इन्सानों के शहर में क्यूँ हैवानियत कर बैठा
कि आइना भी मुझसे आज नाराज़ हो गया है।।

Why did I do an act of the devil in the city of humans
That even the mirror today is upset with me

~

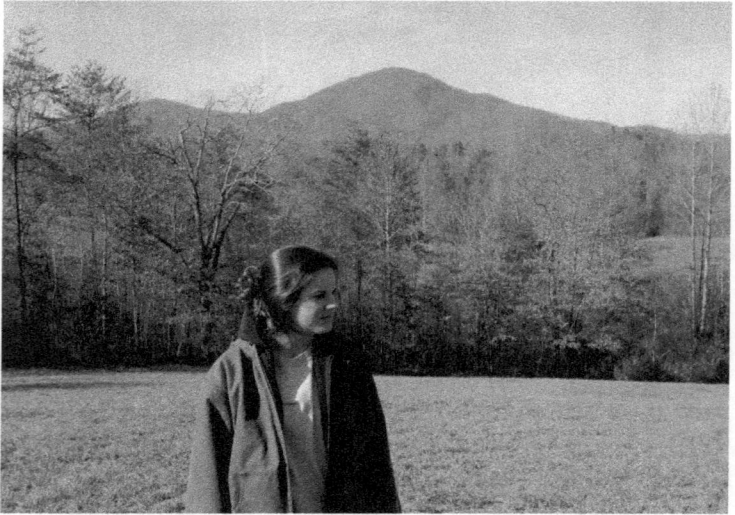

Photograph by Kelly Cameron

कोई कह दो तूफान से मेरा सब्र ना आज़माए
आज राख़ हूँ पर जलाना अब भी जानता हूँ।।

Somebody tell the storm to stop testing my patience
I may be just ash today but I still know how to burn

~

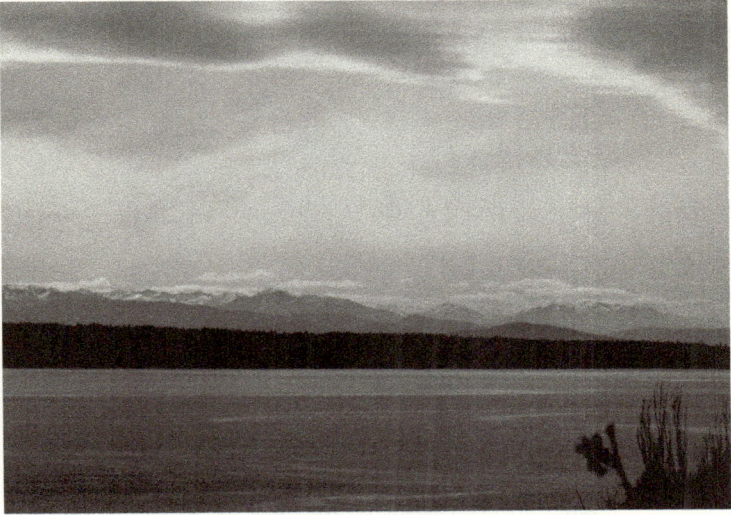

Photograph by Samantha Ehnert

उस सोने का क्या जो सुनहरी रात में सोने ना दे
उस चाँदी का क्या जो चाँद से इश्क होने ना दे
कोई जुगनू-सा मिले और बने फिर हमसफ़र मेरा
तड़पाए सही पर
रात में फिर खोने ना दे।।

What use is that silver that can't let me love the silvery moon
What use is that gold that doesn't let me enjoy the golden rain
I hope a glow-worm I find who becomes my partner in life soon
Who might hide for a while but
won't let me get lost in the dark again

~

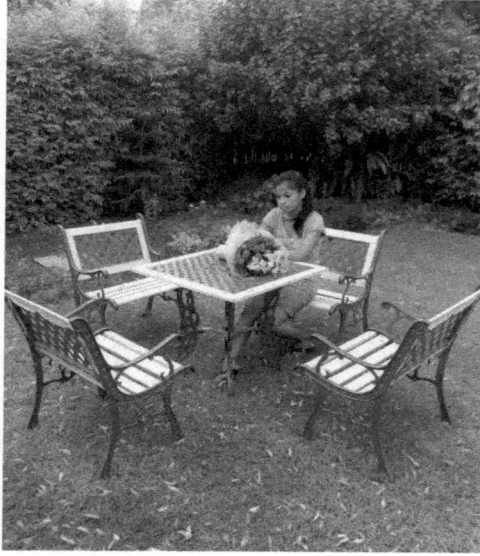

Photograph by Kinshuk Sharma

फूलों का गुलदस्ता नहीं, दिल की धड़कन देना सीखो
फूल तो फूल हैं, समय के साथ मुरझा जाएँगे।।

Learn to give a heartbeat instead of a bouquet of flowers
Flowers are just flowers, with time they'll wither away

~

I've been searching for a while to quench my thirst
But mirage is all I get
The sun used to give me a ray of hope
Today I want it to set

∽

The night was cold, the storm was wild
The dungeon stalled, the blocks were piled
But one I saw, with a lamp of hope
That someone brave, was not a child
Who held that lamp? My wounded heart
Still drenched in hope, like from the start
Though night is dark, still trying to strive
It might not live, but I will survive

～

समय के तराज़ू पे ना तोलो ऐ सनम
मोहब्बत की कश्ती है, मोहब्बत से चलती है।।

Don't measure it on the scale of time, oh love
It's a boat of love, it sails with love

शब्दों की आवाज़ ने कब सच कहा
कागज़ की नमी में असली कविता छुपी है।।

When has the voice of words spoken the truth
Real poetry is hidden in the drop on the page

∼

होंठों पर हँसी से दर्द कब छुपा है
आँखें बंद कर लो, कहीं नज़रें फिर सच ना कह दें।।

When has a smile hidden the pain the heart feels
Close your eyes, they might speak the truth again

~

कोसो ना मय को ऐ हमसफर
नशा तो हम सब में भरा है।।

Don't blame the alcohol, co-traveller
It is us who are really filled with intoxication

~

समुद्री कहर को गलत मत समझना
उसके दिल में मोती अब भी कई हैं।।

Don't misunderstand the wrath of the sea
His heart is still full of pearls of kindness

≈

कुदरत की पलकों पर बिछी है मोती की चादर
लगता है कहीं किसी का दिल आज फिर पिघला है।।

A blanket of pearls decorates the eyelashes of nature
It seems somewhere someone's heart has melted again

~

तेरी आँखों की किताब के वो इश्क वाले पन्ने
कुछ कहानी अधूरी की अधूरी रह गई।।

Those pages of love in the book of your eye
Some parts of the story I just couldn't read

≈

होंठों ने छुआ मय को और तुम दिखे हो
कौन कहता है नशा करना बुरा है।।

Alcohol on my lips and I see you everywhere
Who says intoxication is not a good thing?

~

तूफानों में अँधेरा है या अँधेरे में तूफान
यहाँ चिरागों में चिंगारी भी दिखती नहीं है।।

Is there a dark storm or a storm in the darkness
I can't even see a spark flickering in the lamp

≈

पिघले माणिक की नदी जो दिल से निकलती देखी
उसकी अमीरी की मुझको पहचान हो गई।।

When I saw a river of melted ruby (blood) flowing out
of the heart
I understood why people say that, the heart is priceless

~

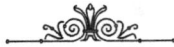

English Songs

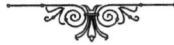

Happiness

In the world of happiness, how did sorrow sink its paws
Things have gone out of way, life has broken its laws
So I sing the merry song, so that people can hear
And I catch the happy notes, so they break through their fears

Because it's the way you look at things, it's an attitude I'd say
I just want to be happy and have fun along the way
I want to send a message down so that people learn it up
Sorrow never did evolve; we poured it in our cup

When I was little, I thought sorrow is in my plate
I'd get some happy days, when I'd be with my mates
But that never occurred, it got worse over time
I looked everywhere, but I didn't hear a chime

Because it's the way you look at things, it's an attitude I'd say
I just want to be happy and have fun along the way
I want to send a message down so that people learn it up
Sorrow never did evolve; we poured it in our cup

I passed my high school days and entered college life
I still couldn't find a thing and thought it'd come with a wife
And now I'm married for over thirty years but still
I've lived a king's life but never got the happy bill

Because it's the way you look at things, it's an attitude I'd say
I just want to be happy and have fun along the way
I want to send a message down so that people learn it up
Sorrow never did evolve; we poured it in our cup

And now I'm about to leave but I do realize a crime
I looked it everywhere, when it was in me all the time
I wasted all my life, searching on a different lane
If you get the right pair of eyes, you would never cry again

Because it's the way you look at things, it's an attitude I'd say
I just want to be happy and have fun along the way
I want to send a message down so that people learn it up
Sorrow never did evolve; we poured it in our cup

≈

Hidden Pain

Your eyes are so numb
Your heart is at stake
You're dropping a smile
But you know it's so fake
You're hitting a low
Your feelings are dry
You're raising the wine
But you're drinking the cry

What are you hiding, why don't you say
The road has been tough but, it's a different day
Oh my love, I care for you
The pain in your heart, gives me a heartache too
What are you hiding, why don't you say
The road has been tough but, it's a different day

A touch of our love
Is a word in your praise
The pain that you feel
Is a passing phase
They say if you share
You're sorrows are halved
You show open field
But the wires are barbed

What are you hiding, why don't you say
The road has been tough but, it's a different day
Oh my love, I care for you
The pain in your heart, gives me a heartache too
What are you hiding, why don't you say
The road has been tough but, it's a different day

It's a different, it's a different, it's a different day
You don't have to walk alone on this road girl
I'm here just for you
To walk you through the day, the night, the love, the fight
Whatever comes by I'm here
Just for you .... (So tell me)

What are you hiding, why don't you say
The road has been tough but, it's a different day
Oh my love, I care for you
The pain in your heart, gives me a heartache too
What are you hiding, why don't you say
The road has been tough but, it's a different day

∿

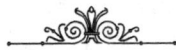

Hindi Songs

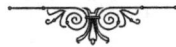

आत्म-हत्या

जान देने से पहले सोचिए इक बात
इन्द्रधनुष क्या बन सके जो ना हो बरसात।।

सूर्य जब यहाँ छुपता है कहीं और सवेरा होता है
नींद ना आए तो कहता दिन को भी वो ढोता है
इक जगह तब बात ना बनी तो बड़ी क्या बात थी
खुशियों की नदी में दो कंकर आ गिरे क्या बात थी
दुख के आँसू से आँखे मींदे
वो होश में बेहोश था
सूर्य के तपस से पूर्व वो नब्ज़ ठँडी कर गया

जाते-जाते यह ना सोचा बाकियों का होगा क्या
दुख तो आते जाते हैं,
दिल के टुकड़ों का होगा क्या।।

साधना में धुत था वो तो
एक जुट भ्रमाँड से
ज़िंदगी की लौ में जलता नीर में बागान में
रात के अँधकार में जलती जो इक मशाल थी
वो जिसे प्रलय था समझा ज़िंदगी की नाव थी
देख भी पाया नहीं वो शोक से मजबूर था
सूर्य के तपस से पूर्व वो नब्ज़ ठँडी कर गया

जाते-जाते यह ना सोचा बाकियों का होगा क्या

दुख तो आते जाते हैं,
दिल के टुकड़ों का होगा क्या।।

खोई थी उसने ज़मीं अब खो दिया है आसमान
वो जिए और हम मरे यह दुख की कैसी दासतान
साथ ना मिल पाए तो तुम सार्थी के साथ हो
कुछ भी ना कर पाए तो तुम कुछ नहीं में खुश रहो
सोचता ना ऐसा उसका जीना तो बेकार था
सूर्य के तपस से पूर्व वो नब्ज़ ठँडी कर गया

जाते-जाते यह ना सोचा बाकियों का होगा क्या
दुख तो आते जाते हैं,
दिल के टुकड़ों का होगा क्या।।

≈

Suicide

Before taking your life, just think this again
Would rainbow be there, if there is no rain

When sun goes down here, it rises to fill someone else's share
If he is not able to sleep properly, he says the day is unfair
If one thing did not go your way, what's the big deal?
If 2 pebbles in river of happiness stay, what's the big deal?
But he was blind with tears so sad
Was out of senses but still not mad
Before he could get the warmth of the sun, he chilled his nerves

He didn't even think what'd happen to his loved ones
Sorrow comes and goes, but
what'd happen to the heart of his loved ones

He was connected with something other than
the world he was in
He used to burn in the fire of life, garden, water and gin
He saw a burning light in the darkness of night
What he thought was a wild fire, was a saviour ship in sight
That sight he could not see , sorrowed eyes are to blame
Before he could get the warmth of the sun, he chilled his nerves

He didn't even think what'd happen to his loved ones

Sorrow comes and goes,
but what'd happen to the heart of his loved ones

He had already lost the land, now he has also lost the sky
He lives and his loved ones die, story of sadness, Why?
If you don't know what to be, let God take care of you
If you can't do a stupid task, maybe you're not meant to
But he didn't think this way because his zest of life was gone
Before he could get the warmth of the sun, he chilled his nerves

He didn't even think what'd happen to his loved ones
Sorrow comes and goes,
but what'd happen to the heart of his loved ones

∾

बातें करे बस नज़र

खयालों से तुम जो हकीकत में आए,
हुआ है यह कैसा असर
खामोश है धड़कन, खामोश है साँसें,
बातें करे बस नज़र।।

इतनी खुशी में हम डूब न जाएँ, बाहों में भर लो पिया
दिल का यह आलम ना लब कह सके पर,
आँखों ने सब कह दिया
आँसू भी रोते, होठों को छूते, ही बोले हैं दिल का हशर
खामोश है धड़कन, खामोश है साँसें,
बातें करे बस नज़र।।

सोचा था हरदम पर कैसे कहें हम, हर पल है चाहा तुम्हें
छुपाए थे दिल में मोहब्बत समन्दर, लहरों से अब ना डरें
आओ हम मिल के इक कश्ती बनाएँ,
शुरू हो सुनहरा सफर
खामोश है धड़कन, खामोश है साँसें,
बातें करे बस नज़र।।

❧

Only Eyes Do the Talking

From dreams that you have come into reality,
Something's happened, don't know how
My heartbeat has stopped, my breath has quietened,
Only eyes do the talking now

I might drown in this happiness, please hug me till I fall
My lips can't say what's going in me, my eyes have said it all
My tears cry too, as they kiss my lips,
What my heart feels is just, Wow!
My heartbeat has stopped, my breath has quietened,
Only eyes do the talking now

I think about how to tell you this, I've loved you all the way
Ocean of love I hid in heart, now I don't fear no bay
Come let us build this boat of love,
To this journey let us bow
My heartbeat has stopped, my breath has quietened,
Only eyes do the talking now

∼

ACKNOWLEDGMENTS

My family, friends and everyone associated with me have played a big role in making me the person I am and encouraging me to write. I want to begin by thanking my parents Sudha and S.M. Sharma, my sisters Garima and Himani, and my brother-in-law Aprameya Kar, who always motivated me to write. They listened to all my poems many times over and sometimes the same ones for days together, just to make me feel good about what I wrote. They helped me write better, gave me suggestions and encouraged me to the point I could take no more. If not for them, I would have never got into writing.

My mentor, Mrs Neena Kumar, who listened to my poems, appreciated them and helped me improve. She taught me the technicalities of different kinds of writing. Saroj aunty, Nirmal uncle and Mrs Susanna Sekely for their encouragement at all times.

Rupa Publications, for making this book a reality.

Last but not the least, my friends Angie Sekely, Kelly Cameron, Samantha Ehnert, Olga Blank, Haley Collins, Alex Whetherell and Liana McHugh, my sister Garima Sharma, and my cousin Varad Tripathi, for their help with the pictures.

www.ingramcontent.com/pod-product-compliance
Lightning Source LLC
Chambersburg PA
CBHW031213270326
41931CB00006B/551